Prostate Cancer Awareness

A Manual for Prostate Cancer Regarding Awareness and Care

Rossana Lewis

TABLE OF CONTENT

Chapter 1: The Function of the Prostate and Potential Complications

First, what is Prostate?

The prostate is a gland below the bladder and in front of the rectum in men and people assigned male at birth (AMAB). It consists of connective tissues and glandular tissues.

Your prostate contributes additional fluid to your semen (ejaculate). Ejaculate is a whitish-gray fluid that releases from your penis when you orgasm. The fluid contains enzymes, zinc and citric acid, which help nourish sperm cells and lubricate your urethra (pronounced "yer-ree-thruh"). The urethra is a tube through which ejaculate and pee flow out of your body.

Your prostate's muscles also help push semen into and through your urethra when you orgasm.

The prostate helps in hormonal metabolism where the male sex testosterone is transformed to a biologically active form, DHT (dihydrotestosterone) and also helps regulate urine flow.

Potential complications of prostate includes:

- **Cancer that spreads (metastasizes):** Prostate cancer can spread to nearby organs, such as your bladder, or travel through your bloodstream or lymphatic system to your bones or other organs. Prostate cancer that spreads to the bones can cause pain and broken bones. Once it has spread to other areas of the body, it may still respond to treatment and may be controlled, but it's unlikely to be cured.

- **Incontinence:** Both prostate cancer and its treatment can cause urinary incontinence. Treatment for incontinence depends on the type you have, how severe it is and the likelihood it will improve over time. Treatment options may include medications, catheters and surgery.

- **Erectile dysfunction:** Erectile dysfunction can result from prostate cancer or its treatment, including surgery, radiation or hormone treatments. Medications, vacuum devices that assist in achieving erection and surgery are available to treat erectile dysfunction.

- **Fatigue:** Treatments like hormone therapy, radiation, and chemotherapy, can make you feel tired. Treatment can also result in low red blood cell counts, which may affect your energy levels.

- **Pain:** Advanced prostate cancer can lead to several types of pain. When it spreads to your bones, you might have bone pain, which often feels like a dull ache. Your tumor may press on a nerve, which could cause a stabbing or burning feeling.

- **Weak bones:** The most common place where prostate cancer spreads is to your bones. In addition to causing pain, this can make them become weak. Hormone therapy can also weaken your bones because it lowers testosterone levels. And weaker bones raise your risk of fractures.

- **Infertility:** You might be unable to father a child through sex.

- **Bladder Damage**: Because the prostate surrounds the urethra and is right next to the bladder, surgery to remove the prostate and its cancer may damage nerves or the bladder outlet muscle (sphincter). This weakens support for the lower bladder and may damage it.

- **Bowel Damage:** Radiotherapy for prostate cancer (external beam radiotherapy and brachytherapy) can cause bowel problems for some men.

Radiation can cause the lining of the bowel to become inflamed (proctitis) which then leads to symptoms such as: loose and watery bowel movements (diarrhea) passing more wind than usual.

Chapter 2. What Triggers Prostate Cancer and How to Avoid it.

It's not known exactly what causes prostate cancer, although a number of things can increase your risk of developing the condition. These include:

Age – the risk rises as you get older, and most cases are diagnosed in men over 50 years of age

Ethnic group – prostate cancer is more common in black men than in Asian men

Family history – having a brother or father who developed prostate cancer before age 60 seems to increase your risk of developing it; research also shows that having a close female relative who developed breast cancer may also increase your risk of developing prostate cancer

Obesity – recent research suggests there may be a link between obesity and prostate cancer, and a balanced diet and regular exercise may lower your risk of developing prostate cancer

Diet – research is ongoing into the links between diet and prostate cancer, and there is some evidence that a diet high in calcium is linked to an increased risk of developing prostate cancer.

Improve Your Diet

Researchers don't completely understand the relationship between diet and prostate cancer prevention, but studies suggest that certain eating habits may help.

- **Reduce fat intake:** Eat less trans fats and saturated fats. Focus on healthy fats such as omega-3 fatty acids from nuts, seeds and fish.

- **Eat more fruits and vegetables**. Incorporate a wide variety of produce, including plenty of leafy greens. The antioxidant lycopene, which is plentiful in cooked or processed tomatoes, has been shown in some studies to slow the growth of prostate cancer cells. Cruciferous vegetables (e.g., broccoli and cauliflower) contain a compound called sulforaphane that may protect against cancer.

- **Add green tea and soy**: Clinical trials have suggested that soy may lower PSA levels, and that green tea may help men who are at high risk for prostate cancer lower their risk.

- **Avoid charred meat**: Charred meat, from frying or grilling at high temperatures, may produce a chemical compound that leads to cancer.

Other things apart from improved diet that may be considered are:

- **Maintaining Healthy Weight:** Obesity can be a risk factor for developing more aggressive prostate cancer. In general, losing weight and maintaining a healthy weight as you age can help reduce your risk of cancer and many other health problems.

- **Get Regular Exercise:** In addition to helping you achieve a healthy weight, exercise can reduce inflammation, improve immune function and fight some of the negative health effects of a sedentary lifestyle—all of which can help prevent cancer.

- **Stop Smoking and Drink Less:** Quitting smoking can improve your health in many ways, including lowering your cancer risk. And if you drink, do so in moderation. Some studies suggest that red wine has antioxidant properties that may benefit your health.

- **Increase Your Vitamin D:** Most people don't get enough vitamin D. It can help protect against prostate cancer and many other conditions. Vitamin D-rich foods include cod liver oil, wild salmon and dried shiitake mushrooms. Since the sun is a better, more readily available source of vitamin D, many experts recommend getting 10 minutes of sun exposure (without sunscreen) every day. Doctors often recommend vitamin D supplements. However, you should talk to your doctor before taking any vitamins or supplements.

- **Stay Sexually Active:** Two studies appear to show that men who have a higher frequency of ejaculation (with or without a sexual partner) were up to two-thirds less likely to be diagnosed with prostate cancer. Studies are ongoing, but some experts theorize that ejaculation clears the body of toxins and other substances that could cause inflammation.

Chapter 3: Is there Prostate Cancer in me? Identification and Examination

As prostate cancer rarely produces symptoms in its early stages, there are a few signs that may signal something is wrong in the prostate.

Here are five potential warning signs of prostate cancer:

- A painful or burning sensation during urination or ejaculation
- Frequent urination, particularly at night
- Difficulty stopping or starting urination
- Sudden erectile dysfunction
- Blood in urine or semen

Other possible early signs of prostate cancer include unusually weak urine flow and unexplained pain around the prostate while sitting. If cancer has spread beyond the prostate gland, men may experience swelling in the lower body, back, hip or bone pain, abnormal bowel or urinary habits or unexplained weight loss.

It is important to note that the signs of prostate cancer are also shared by many other, less-serious conditions. If you are displaying one or more of these symptoms, it does not necessarily mean that you have prostate cancer. Similarly, a man who is diagnosed with prostate cancer may not have any of these symptoms.

Cancer examination means looking for cancer before it causes symptoms. The goal of screening for prostate cancer is to find cancers that may be at high risk for spreading if not treated, and to find them early before they spread.

If you are thinking about being screened, learn about the possible benefits and harms of screening, diagnosis, and treatment, and talk to your doctor about your personal risk factors.

There is no standard test to screen for prostate cancer. Two tests that are commonly used to screen for prostate cancer are described below:

Prostate Specific Antigen (PSA) Test

A blood test called a prostate specific antigen (PSA) test measures the level of PSA in the blood. PSA is a substance made by the prostate. The levels of PSA in the blood can be higher in men who have prostate cancer. The PSA level may also be elevated in other conditions that affect the prostate.

As a rule, the higher the PSA level in the blood, the more likely a prostate problem is present. But many factors, such as age and race, can affect PSA levels. Some prostate glands make more PSA than others.

PSA levels also can be affected by—

- Certain medical procedures.
- Certain medications.
- An enlarged prostate.
- A prostate infection.

Because many factors can affect PSA levels, your doctor is the best person to interpret your PSA test results. If the PSA test is abnormal, your doctor may recommend a biopsy to find out if you have prostate cancer.

Digital Rectal Examination (DRE)

Digital rectal examination (DRE) is when a health care provider inserts a gloved, lubricated finger into a man's rectum to feel the prostate for anything abnormal, such as cancer. The U.S Preventive Services Task Force does not recommend DRE as a screening test because of lack evidence on the benefits.

Chapter 4: Assessment and Staging

When a digital rectal exam (DRE) or a PSA test reveal abnormal results, the next step is further testing to determine whether prostate cancer is present, or another cause may be to blame.

Your doctor will evaluate your test results and any symptoms you may be experiencing and recommend the next tests you may need. The most common diagnostic tests for the prostate include:

1. Ultrasound: A transrectal ultrasound involves inserting a small ultrasound probe into the rectum. The ultrasound machine sends out sound waves and then measures the "echoes" that bounce back off body structures to create an image of

the "landscape" of the structure. It can provide images that show the extent of prostate enlargement or abnormalities.

2. MRI: Magnetic resonance imaging (MRI) is sometimes used to create a more detailed set of images than an ultrasound can provide. Results will be reported as a PI-RADS score.

- PI-RADS 1: very low—clinically significant cancer is highly unlikely to be present

- PI-RADS 2: low—clinically significant cancer is unlikely to be present

- PI-RADS 3: intermediate—the chance of clinically significant cancer is neutral

- PI-RADS 4: high—clinically significant cancer is likely to be present

- PI-RADS 5: very high—clinically significant cancer is highly likely to be present

3. Biopsy: A biopsy entails taking a sample of tissue for examination under a microscope. A biopsy can be taken via a needle or needles inserted into the prostate, or a larger sample can be obtained surgically (anesthesia is used, and your doctor will offer you appropriate pain relief). Often, ultrasound is used to guide the needles to the exact area of concern. Biopsy technology is advancing quickly and can be combined with imaging techniques to increase accuracy:

- TRUS-guided biopsy: A trans-rectal ultrasound–guided biopsy is the most common way prostate cancer is diagnosed in the US. An ultrasound probe is placed in the rectum to allow visualization of the prostate. Then at least 12 needles are placed into the prostate to take samples that are examined for abnormal cells. (Twelve needles sounds like a lot, but the more varied the sample, the greater the chance of catching any abnormal cells.) If a patient had magnetic resonance imaging (MRI) before the biopsy, the MRI images may help target areas that looked suspicious.

- Trans-perineal biopsy: A biopsy sample can also be obtained by placing a needle through the perineum, the skin between the scrotum and anus.

4. Incidental procedures: Sometimes, doctors performing surgery in a nearby area actually see something amiss with the

prostate and can take a sample during the same procedure.

Regardless of which procedure is used to take a sample, the prostate tissue is then examined under a microscope by a pathologist, to confirm the presence or absence of cancerous cells.

Biopsy technology continues to improve. New research is isolating better and better ways to increase accuracy of biopsies to zero in on problem areas and achieve the goal of a minimally-invasive biopsy procedure that has the greatest chance of sampling cells, with minimal damage to surrounding tissues. Targeted, or fusion biopsies are increasingly being utilized at select centers that use an MRI, in addition to the ultrasound, to better visualize tumors within the prostate and help guide biopsy needles.

Now, let's talk about the staging of this ailment. A cancer's stage is an assessment that takes into account a variety of factors: the cancer's location, whether it has spread, or metastasized, and how much it's interfering with normal body processes.

Generally, the stage of a person's cancer is correlated with their chances for survival. But it's important to understand that different types of cancer have very different treatment success rates. Some types of cancer are highly treatable, and even patients diagnosed at stage IV can reasonably expect their treatment will be successful. Other types of cancer are very resistant to treatment, and even patients diagnosed at lower stages are in for a very tough fight. Prostate cancer is often highly treatable.

If your doctors confirm that you have prostate cancer, they will begin a process of assessing several factors to determine your stage. This will help them recommend the best possible treatments, customized for you.

There are 4 main components to staging prostate cancer:

- Your PSA level
- The grade of your tumor (done via biopsy)
- The stage of your tumor (termed the T-stage for the prostate tumor)—for example, is the prostate cancer contained completely within the prostate?
- Whether the cancer has spread, or metastasized, to lymph nodes (termed the "N-stage" for nodes) or bones or other organs (termed the "M-stage" for metastasis).

Chapter 5: What Choices Do I have

When diagnosed with prostate cancer, you may have several thoughts considering the treatment suitable. There are three major treatment options: Active Surveillance, surgery, and radiation therapy. For patients whose cancer appears more aggressive, combination treatment may be recommended. For example, radiation therapy may be combined with hormone therapy, and surgery may be followed by radiation, sometimes with the addition of hormone therapy.

Choosing the best treatment for localized or locally advanced prostate cancer is generally based on age, the stage and grade of the cancer, the patient's general health, and an evaluation of the risks and benefits of each therapy option.

Health care providers think about localized or locally advanced prostate cancer in terms of "risk groups," which are assigned before the patient undergoes any treatment. There are 3 general risk groups based on the PSA, DRE, and biopsy, which can further be subdivided to better personalize treatment for each patient.

The treatment options for each risk group have some differences; ask your doctor which risk group you belong to so you can better understand the most appropriate next steps.

For active surveillance for prostate cancer, your prostate cancer is closely monitored for any changes. Active surveillance for prostate cancer is sometimes called expectant management.

No cancer treatment is provided during active surveillance for prostate cancer. This means medications, radiation and surgery aren't used. Periodic tests are done to check for signs the cancer is growing. You might consider active surveillance for prostate cancer if your cancer is small, expected to grow very slowly, confined to one area of your prostate, and isn't causing signs or symptoms. If you have other health problems that limit your life expectancy, active surveillance for prostate cancer may also be a reasonable approach.

Surgery for prostate cancer involves removing the prostate gland (radical prostatectomy), some surrounding tissue and a few lymph nodes. Surgery is an option for treating cancer that's confined to the prostate. It's sometimes used to treat advanced prostate cancer in combination with other treatments. To access the prostate, surgeons may use a technique that involves:

- Making several small incisions in your abdomen. During robot-assisted laparoscopic prostatectomy, surgical instruments are attached to a mechanical device (robot) and inserted through several small incisions in your abdomen. The surgeon sits at a console and uses hand controls to guide the robot to move the instruments. Most prostate cancer operations are done using this technique.

- Making one long incision in your abdomen. During retropubic surgery, the surgeon makes one long incision in your lower abdomen to access and remove the prostate gland. This approach is much less common, but may be necessary in certain situations.

For radiation therapy, high-powered energy is used to kill cancer cells. Prostate cancer radiation therapy treatments may involve:

- Radiation that comes from outside of your body (external beam radiation). During external beam radiation therapy, you lie on a table while a machine moves around your body, directing high-powered energy beams, such as X-rays or protons, to your prostate cancer. You typically undergo external beam radiation treatments five days a week for several weeks. Some medical centers offer a shorter course of radiation therapy that uses higher doses of radiation spread over fewer days. External beam radiation is an option for treating cancer that's confined to the prostate. It can also be used after surgery to kill any cancer cells that might remain if there's a risk that the cancer could spread or come back. For prostate cancer that spreads to other areas of the body, such as the bones, radiation therapy can help slow the cancer's growth and relieve symptoms, such as pain.

- Radiation placed inside your body (brachytherapy). Brachytherapy involves placing radioactive sources in your prostate tissue. Most often, the radiation is contained in rice-sized radioactive seeds that are inserted into your prostate tissue. The seeds deliver a low dose of radiation over a long period of time. Brachytherapy is one option for treating cancer that hasn't spread beyond the prostate.

In some situations, doctors may recommend both types of radiation therapy.

Chapter 6: Sexual Minorities in Prostate Cancer

Patients with prostate cancer from sexual minority groups experience considerably worse quality of life following prostate cancer treatment than heterosexual patients. Improved inclusivity as well as cultural humility training at the physician, institution and system levels are warranted to address inequalities in quality-of-life outcomes.

Prostate cancer is the second most common malignancy among men across the world, with 1,414,259 estimated patients in 2020 alone1. Despite the high global incidence of this disease, treatment patterns for prostate cancer as well as short-term and long-term effects of treatment in patients remain poorly understood in sexual and gender minority groups including gay and bisexual men (GBM) and transgender women. Sexual and gender minority groups have historically encountered a multitude of challenges when navigating traditionally heteronormative health-care systems to seek cancer care; obstacles include lack of medical insurance owing to discrimination in obtaining jobs, lack of comfort in sharing sexual orientation with the treating physician, lack of inclusive training received by physicians, lack of available support groups for patients and lack of (or diminished) social support systems from long-term partners and family. A growing recognition of this 'hidden population' emerged over the past decade; thus, several qualitative studies and a limited number of quantitative works have been undertaken to have an improved understanding of the effects of prostate cancer treatment on quality of life in patients from sexual and gender minority groups.

Prostate Cancer Treatment in Sexual Minorities

Treatment options for localized prostate cancer include external beam radiation therapy (RT) with or without brachytherapy, brachytherapy alone, radical prostatectomy, or active surveillance. These options are recommended based on the risk stratifications provided by the American Society of Clinical Oncology, American Urological Association, American Society for Radiation Oncology, and Society of Urologic Oncology. The decision regarding treatment is arrived at after a discussion with the patient, weighing the potential risks against the benefits. A study utilizing an online prostate cancer discussion board demonstrated that gay men were more worried about the negative impacts of treatment and the availability of psychological and emotional support, whereas straight men were more interested in exploring the different treatment options available to them. These concerns by gay men may impact treatment preferences, but additional research is required to substantiate this possibility.

It is unclear if treatment patterns in the GBM community differ from heterosexual men. For example, there have been reports that Gleason scores were found to be significantly lower in GBM treated for prostate cancer than in heterosexual men. In a study performed by Murphy in Chicago, it was found that men who are HIV-positive are equally likely to receive treatment for prostate cancer. However, they are less likely to undergo a radical prostatectomy and more likely to receive overtreatment compared to men who are HIV-negative. Use of ARV treatment for HIV has been suggested to be protective in prostate cancer.

A study included 460 heterosexual and 92 non-heterosexual men in their study and they observed no difference in treatment pattern between heterosexual and non-heterosexual. In a study by Hart et al., it was found that the rates of prostatectomy, external beam radiation, and ADT in gay men were 55.4%, 27.2%, and 25%, respectively. While there was no control group of heterosexual men included in the study, the rates of treatment choices in gay men were similar to those observed in the general population. Another cross-sectional study with a cohort of gay men, which also lacked a heterosexual control group, found that these men had slightly higher rates of surgical treatment (60.4%) and similar rates of radiotherapy (27%) compared to the general population. Ussher et al. found in their study that gay and bisexual men were slightly less likely to receive radiotherapy than heterosexual men. Although these studies provide some understanding of the patterns in treatments, they do not explain the decision-making process involved in treatment or how this varies between heterosexual and non-heterosexual men.

Clinical Implications and Future Directions
By delving into the specifics of prostate cancer screening, diagnosis, treatment, and quality of life, healthcare professionals can offer more culturally appropriate care to their patients. Nonetheless, further research is necessary to

explore how prostate cancer impacts sexual minority groups in various ethnicities, cultures, and regions worldwide, as most of the data presented in this review originates from studies conducted in European and North American countries. We have highlighted the nuances of prostate cancer treatment and its impact on the quality of life of sexual minority patients. Nevertheless, additional studies are needed to guide the nursing and supportive care of sexual minorities following prostate cancer treatment.

Chapter 7: Success Rate for Treating Localized Prostate Cancer

There are different types of statistics that can help doctors evaluate a person's chance of recovery from prostate cancer. These are called survival statistics. A specific type of survival statistic is called the relative survival rate. It is often used to predict how having cancer may affect life expectancy. Relative survival rate looks at how likely people with prostate cancer are to survive for a certain amount of time after their initial diagnosis or start of treatment compared to the expected survival of similar people without this cancer.

It is important to remember that statistics on the survival rates for people with prostate cancer are only an estimate. They cannot tell an individual if cancer will or will not shorten their life. Instead, these statistics describe trends in groups of people previously diagnosed with the same disease, including specific stages of the disease.

The 5-year relative survival rate for prostate cancer in the United States is 97%. The 10-year relative survival rate is 98%.

The survival rates for prostate cancer vary based on several factors. These include the stage and grade of the cancer, a person's age and general health, and how well the treatment plan works. Another factor that can affect outcomes is the type of prostate cancer.

Approximately 83% of prostate cancers are found when the disease is in only the prostate and nearby organs (70% local and 13% regional). This is referred to as the local or regional stage. The 5-year relative survival rate for most people with local or regional prostate cancer is nearly 100%. For people diagnosed with prostate cancer that has spread to other parts of the body, the 5-year relative survival rate is 32%.

Experts measure relative survival rate statistics for prostate cancer every 5 years. This means the estimate may not reflect the results of advancements in how prostate cancer is diagnosed or treated from the last 5 years. Talk with your doctor if you have any questions about this information.

Chapter 8: Erectile Problems Following Localized Cancer Therapy

About 25 to 50% of men who undergo brachytherapy will experience erectile dysfunction vs. nearly 50% of men who have standard external beam radiation. After two to three years, few men will see much of an improvement and occasionally these numbers worsen over time.

Men who undergo procedures not designed to minimize side effects and/or those whose treatments are administered by physicians who are not proficient in the procedures will fare worse.

Men with other diseases or disorders that impair their ability to maintain an erection (diabetes, vascular problems, etc.) will have a more difficult time returning to pre-treatment function. Prostate cancer can possibly damage the nerves that control these erections and can lower the testosterone level which can in turn cause erectile dysfunction after treatment.

Management of Erectile Dysfunction

Oral medications relax the muscles in the penis, allowing blood to rapidly flow in. On average, the drugs take about an hour to begin working, and the erection-helping effects can last from 8 to 36 hours.

About 75% of men who undergo nerve-sparing prostatectomy or more precise forms of radiation therapy have reported successfully achieving erections after using these drugs. However, they are not for everyone, including men who take medications for angina or other heart problems and men who take alpha-blockers.

Chapter 9: Therapy with Hormones/Androgen

Hormone therapy is also called androgen suppression therapy. The goal of this treatment is to reduce levels of male hormones, called androgens, in the body, or to stop them from fueling prostate cancer cell growth.

Androgens stimulate prostate cancer cells to grow. The main androgens in the body are testosterone and dihydrotestosterone (DHT). Most androgens are made by the testicles, but the adrenal glands (glands that sit above your kidneys) as well as the prostate cancer cells themselves, can also make androgens.

Lowering androgen levels or stopping them from getting into prostate cancer cells often makes prostate cancers shrink or grow more slowly for a time. But hormone therapy alone does not cure prostate cancer.

When is hormone therapy used?

Hormone therapy may be used:

- If the cancer has spread too far to be cured by surgery or radiation, or if you can't have these treatments for some other reason

- If the cancer remains or comes back after treatment with surgery or radiation therapy

- Along with radiation therapy as the initial treatment, if you are at higher risk of the cancer coming back after treatment (based on a high Gleason score, high PSA level, and/or growth of the cancer outside the prostate).

- Before radiation to try to shrink the cancer to make treatment more effective

Away from this book, it would be really appreciated if you could provide a review if you thought it was worthwhile as it would motivate me. Thanks.